Diabetes

Best Drug Free Guide to Reverse Diabetes and Lower Blood Sugar

Disclaimer

The author is not a doctor. Anyone who has diabetes should seek immediate help from a doctor. Nobody should ever stop taking their prescription diabetic medications cold turkey. If a person has diabetes and is under the care of a doctor, that person can then, under their doctor's supervision, try to gradually wean themselves off of prescriptions drugs and regain their health through weight loss, diet and exercise. A person who does not yet have diabetes may be able to prevent themselves from getting the disease, but the author makes no promises. The author does not accept responsibility for adverse results that may stem from what readers of this book do with the information in it.

Table of Contents

Introduction

Congratulations on downloading this book and thank you for doing so.

It only takes a few key lifestyle changes to avoid diabetes. These same few lifestyle changes may even take you back out of a diabetic's life, away from that life you now lead...sticking yourself to test your blood, enduring frequent half-days at your local dialysis center, evenings spent waiting in line at the pharmacy, and/or foot amputation.

In Western society, we have veered off of doing the three things that would keep diabetes and the miseries that are associated with it out of our future. Those three things are keeping the weight off, a healthy diet, and getting enough exercise.

These things sound boring and possibly even dreadful to many of us, but it is better to fit these things into our lives now than to spend our old age dealing with diabetes. And if there is a way to reverse diabetes in a person who already has this disease, this healthy lifestyle would obviously be the way.

Our modern ways of eating are a far cry from how our ancestors ate. We have replaced pure and fresh homegrown, home-cooked square meals that include lots of fruit and vegetables with drive-through burgers, boxed dinners, and other commercially made unhealthy food that leave us fat and generally unhealthy through the years.

With cars and other modern forms of transportation, exercise is an activity that most of us in Western society don't do enough of. Walking a mile or two a day to get somewhere and another mile or two just in the process of doing daily work or chores is just no longer part of life for many Americans.

Between bad diets and little exercise, we end up getting fat, and obesity is the number one risk to getting diabetes. To many of us in today's age, looking good and attractive to the opposite sex is a distant memory by the time we reach middle age. We remain fat through the years and then end up with diabetes or one of the other big diseases later on in life. We consider it all to be normal, though, telling ourselves that all of this is just part of getting old.

With the cost of healthcare getting out of reach financially, however, people are becoming desperate for answers. People wonder whether they can actually control or even reverse this dreadful disease through the natural remedies.

This book will tell you specific changes to your lifestyle that you need to make so as to keep diabetes out of your future and to possibly even reverse the disease if you currently have it.

Weight loss in general needs to be taken off, but there is one area of the body that puts people at the most risk of getting diabetes. That particular area of the body is discussed in this book, as are the particular foods one needs to avoid eating so as to keep the weight off of that area.

You will learn about the specific powerful wild plants that you can grow in your own pharmaceutical garden and then include in your diet to avoid, manage and hopefully even reverse diabetes. Throw them into salads or include them with other fresh produce when you make smoothies.

Form new habits. Change your future. Watch your health and life change in just a short while. Get this book and find out how.

The following chapters will include a brief discussion about what diabetes is so that all readers know exactly what the disease is. Lifestyle changes that all diabetics and "pre-diabetics" need to make will be the focus of this book.

Weight loss, a proper diet, and physical exercise are universally understood to be the areas in which lifestyle changes need to be made if one is going to address diabetes.

This book, however, adds a hefty section that describes the powerful edible plants that often get omitted in discussions about diabetes. These include berries, flowers, grass, herbs, seaweed, tree nuts and other things from nature. It is the author's view that we can make a difference in our health by going back to eating as nature intended. Extra care of feet needs to be taken too if one is diabetic, so there is a chapter about foot care included.

These changes could seem daunting at first, depending on how far away from nature one has strayed, but making the needed changes does not have to be feared. New habits can be formed in these areas as they are in any other area. Plan your meals and make the grocery lists to support them. In time, you will know what you need at the store without consulting a list.

This book was written so that you can prevent yourself from getting diabetes if you don't yet have it. It was also written for diabetics to help them manage or perhaps even reverse the disease.

There are many books on this subject on the market. Thanks again for choosing this one! Every effort was made to ensure it is full of as much useful information as possible. Please enjoy!

Chapter 1: About Diabetes

Definition

Diabetes is actually a group of metabolic diseases that feature prolonged high blood sugar levels.

Cause of Diabetes

For a person to get diabetes, either the cells of the body do not respond properly to insulin, or else the pancreas is not producing enough insulin.

Types of Diabetes

Type 1 diabetes mellitus is the kind that people are born with and is the kind when the pancreas just doesn't produce enough insulin.

Type 2 diabetes mellitus is the kind that people contract when their cells stop responding to insulin the way they should, and it sometimes progresses until their bodies won't make insulin. Excessive weight and lack of exercise are usually the causes of this one, along with a poor diet.

Gestational diabetes is short-term. It occurs when a pregnant woman develops a high sugar level who didn't have high sugar levels before she was pregnant.

Some people now argue that dementia is diabetes of the brain, which is a concept that is currently under study. Dementia may one day be considered the fourth type of diabetes.

Symptoms

High blood sugar levels cause increased thirst, increased hunger, and frequent urination.

Acute Complications

Acute complications of diabetes include diabetic nonketotic hyperosmolar coma, ketoacidosis, or death.

Serious Long-Term Complications

Heart disease, chronic kidney failure, stroke, damage to eyes and foot ulcers are complications that are possible long-term complications that can come about as a result of diabetes.

Chapter 2: Prevent/Treat/Reverse Diabetes with Weight Loss

Obesity is the number one risk factor for getting Type 2 diabetes so it would be reasonable to assume that getting rid of it weight would not only help to prevent getting the disease but might also help to reverse the condition.

Fortunately, weight loss comes naturally through proper diet and adequate exercise. There is one aspect of obesity that does need to be specifically addressed, however, and that is the location of the body that one packs it on.

A Bloated Abdomen…the Biggest Diabetic Risk

Have you seen women who look pregnant all the time but aren't? They carry weight in the abdomen. Sometimes you see men carry weight below the belly button and it looks a bit odd on a man. These people are at high risk for getting diabetes.

A person may be heavy, but the risk of getting diabetes gets even higher if that person carries extra weight in the abdomen area. Belly fat surrounds the liver and other abdominal organs that are closely linked to insulin resistance.

Avoid fructose-laden food to help flatten the abdomen. Calories that come from fructose are more likely than any other substance to add weight to your abdomen. If you want to get that tummy flat and keep yourself away from a life with diabetes, you need to avoid these like the plague.

You should avoid the following items:

- Soda
- Energy drinks
- Sports drinks
- Coffee drinks

Also stay away from processed foods such as:

- Doughnuts
- Candy
- Muffins
- Cereal
- Granola bars

Flush old fecal matter out of your colon to help flatten the abdomen. Here is a health and beauty secret that you won't find a lot of people in Western society discussing, but that doesn't make it unimportant. And if you want to get that abdomen much flatter immediately, getting you off to an encouraging start to a new way of living, colonics will do it.

Almost everybody is carrying around at least a few pounds of old fecal matter in their colon, which accumulates over time if it is not regularly flushed out through a lifetime of healthy eating or else through frequent colonics or enemas.

There are various estimates as to how much old fecal matter that actor John Wayne had in his gut when he died, but one person estimated it to be about 75 pounds. Why let that junk stay in there like he did? Get it out.

It will take many sessions to get it all out if you have a lot of it packed in there. Sessions are expensive and humiliating to have done by somebody else so it would be worth it to invest in your own system that you do at home in the privacy of your own bathroom.

Once the old fecal matter is off of the walls of your colon, your body will start to absorb nutrients better, and you will immediately feel cleaner, lighter, sexier, more energetic, and your mood and outlook will improve.

Flush out candida or parasite overgrowth to start ridding self of the cause of sugar cravings that keep your abdomen fat. If you have an overgrowth of candida or parasites, they could be big you are obese and carry weight around the abdomen.

Flushing out the old pipes with water will give you a jump start on evacuating the little critters. You can read up a little more on getting rid of candida and parasites in chapter 3 in the section that talks about sugar cravings and then do research if you want to know more about these subjects. We won't go into detail about either one of those subjects here, though.

Not only is sugar addictive, but if you are hosting a lot of candida or parasite, they are a whole lot of the reason for your chronic need for lots of sugar. If you crave the sugary food that is listed above, which forces your body to carry weight around the abdomen, you need to do whatever it takes to help yourself to succeed in your battle against diabetes.

Chapter 3: Prevent/Treat/Reverse Diabetes with Food

People who have diabetes are at almost twice the risk of getting heart disease as the general population. Mental health problems also increase in diabetics. There is good news, though, because Type 2 diabetes is preventable in most cases, and it can even be reversed in some cases by taking the proper steps that are necessary for diet, weight loss, and exercise.

People ask themselves, "What can I eat?" There is no need to feel deprived. You just need to make different food choices than you are used to making for the majority of what you consume. After that, it becomes a habit.

The biggest food factor for addressing diabetes is the carbohydrates that a person eats. There are good sources and bad sources of carbs, and which ones you eat on a regular basis make a big difference in your ability to manage your diabetes.

A Mediterranean style of diet is a healthy and tasty way to eat if you are diabetic or are wanting to avoid becoming diabetic. Of course, there are other heart-healthy kinds of food one can eat.

Making a shopping list with particular meals in mind is a good idea. Having quick, healthy snack options available at all times is also a good idea.

Let's get some of the myths about a diabetic's food options out of the way and then go on to the meat of the information concerning one's ideal diet.

Myths

Myth: You must cut out all sugar.
Fact: You just need to plan for it and limit the hidden sugar in store-bought food.

Myth: You must cut out most carbohydrates.
Fact: You just need to eat certain types of carbohydrates and watch the serving size of it.

Myth: You must eat special diabetic meals.
Fact: You are just eating healthy. Additionally, there is no need to spend a lot of money on what is advertised as diabetic food.

Myth: You need a high-protein diet.
Fact: Too much protein, especially from animal sources, may cause insulin resistance. Insulin resistance is a key factor in diabetes. We all need protein, carbohydrates, and fats in our diets.

Eat More

-   Healthy fats – olive oil, fish oils, nuts, flax seeds and avocados
-   Vegetables and fruits – whole fruit rather than juices, and lots of fresh, colorful non-starchy vegetables
-   High fiber whole grain or legume cereals, such as bran flakes, bread, and pasta
-   Brown rice
-   Shellfish and fish plus organic turkey or chicken
-   High-quality protein – eggs, beans, unsweetened yogurt and low-fat dairy
-   Steel-cut or rolled oats

Eat Less

-   Trans fats from deep-fried food or partially hydrogenated food
-   Fast food and packaged food, especially chips and food that is high in sugar, such   as baked goods, desserts, and other sweets
-   White bread, white rice, refined pasta or sugary cereals
-   Red meat, processed meat
-   Low-fat food items such as fat-free yogurt that replaced fat with sugar
-   Instant oatmeal

Carbohydrates

Don't let people fool you when they tell you that you need to give up all carbohydrates because that is not the case. You may just need to switch out what it is that you are eating most often for carbs to the healthier versions and then keep all carbohydrates under 120 grams daily.

You need to eat carbohydrates that are high-fiber, slow-release carbohydrates so that sugar is released into your blood at a slower rate. Limit refined carbohydrates such as white bread, white rice, pasta, candy, soda, snacks and packaged meals.

It might seem that since carbohydrates have the biggest effect on blood sugar levels that a diet that is low in carbohydrates would benefit diabetics. A low-carb diet is beneficial when you are talking about cutting way down on things like sugar and white bread. Weight loss would be quick, and blood sugar could be better managed if you cut those items out of the diet.

Eat the good carbs, though, because the glucose those carbs create fuel your brain. Your brain can get fuel from protein and fat if you eat truly low carb food, say 20 to 50 grams of carbohydrates per day, but that would produce large amounts of harmful ketones. You need to keep your carbohydrate intake closer to 120 grams per day. That is enough to fuel your brain, yet low enough to not upset your blood glucose level.

The Atkins diet has been telling people to eat almost no carbohydrates but lots of bacon, hamburger, etc. People have had mixed results, but the fact is that more food that contains saturated fat is consumed on that diet. That increases the risk for cancer and heart disease. Other low-carb fad diets have emerged that tell people to cut out whole grains, fruit, and starchy vegetables.

While the American Diabetes Association doesn't advocate for or against low-carb plans, it should be noted that if a person who is on insulin suddenly restricts their carb intake, that person's blood glucose will drop.

People who are against a low-carb diet say that almost nobody can keep up a strict no-carb or low-carb diet over a long period of time. One needs the fiber of carb-rich food such as whole grains and beans to keep regular, not constipated. Elimination of carbs from the diet also leads to fatigue and foggy thinking.

Most of the experts who advocate a low-carb diet suggest eating lots of non-starchy vegetables and salads with healthy fats, and lean protein sources instead of the bacon free-for-all of the Atkins diet. They argue that people who do not consume many carbs at all can lower their insulin dose, which reduces their risk for hypoglycemia.

One diabetic who only consumed 30 grams per day of carbs said that his blood glucose and the cholesterol improved so much that he was taken off of their Metformin and cholesterol medication.

The arguments go both ways. If you do plan to make a switch to an extremely low-carb diet like that, you need to talk it over with your doctor and make a plan. You don't want to have a sudden drop-off of blood glucose when you are on medication. Check your levels often and consult your doctor regularly.

Glycemic Index

Foods that have a high glycemic index spike your blood sugar level quickly. Using this index to manage blood sugar is often promoted, but it is not without some drawbacks. Those drawbacks include:
-    The benefits of using the glycemic index are unclear.
-    Referring to the index is complicated.
-    The index does not measure the healthfulness of the food.
-    Research shows the Mediterranean or other diets that are good for the heart will help you to lower your glycemic index and improve the quality of your diet.

Cut out Extra Sugar

- Slowly reduce your cravings by slowly removing sugar from your diet.
- If you want dessert, forego the bread, rice and/or pasta during the meal.
- Eat healthy fat so that sugars don't spike as quickly. We're talking about nuts, yogurt, ricotta cheese, peanut butter, etc.
- Sweets eaten by themselves cause sugar to spike, so eat them with the other food.
- Savor your food instead of gulping everything down quickly.
- Reduce the number of soft drinks you intake.
- Don't substitute sugar in place of saturated fat as is the case with refined carbs and whole milk. Watch what was substituted when an item is marked as "low fat.
- Sweeten your food yourself. Buy plain yogurt and unsweetened tea, etc.,   because you will likely add less sugar than the manufacturers would.
- Check the labels to find the low-sugar products. Go for fresh/frozen options rather than canned.
- Avoid packaged or processed foods such as frozen dinners, canned soup or   low-fat meals
- Use less sugar in recipes and boost sweetness with nutmeg, vanilla extract,   mint, or cinnamon.
- Find healthier ways to satisfy your need for sweets. Make frozen banana shakes. Eat some dark chocolate instead of milk chocolate.
- Give yourself half of the dessert size you would normally take, then put fruit in place of the missing half.
- Don't underestimate the carbohydrates and calories in alcoholic drinks.

Hidden Sugar

Be aware that sugar is being put into all sorts of food that it should not be in, such as fast food meals, many packaged meals, staples such as instant mashed potatoes, ketchup, low-fat meals, frozen dinners, margarine, pasta sauce, bread, canned goods, and cereal.

Some ingredients on labels are more obvious than others about being sugar. Manufacturers are sneaky, putting sources of sugar in their food from different sources and from so many sources scattered down a list that it is difficult to see how much sugar is actually in a product. Know what they are and then add them up and you will get a good idea of how much sugar is actually in the food you are considering buying. Anything that ends with "ose," for instance, is a dead give-away that it is a type of sugar.

Memorize and try to avoid the following sources of added sugar:

- Sugar
- Honey
- Molasses
- Malt syrup
- Maltose
- Lactose
- Evaporated cane juice
- Invert sugar
- Fructose
- High-fructose corn syrup
- Dextrose
- Crystalline fructose
- Corn sweetener
- Cane crystals,
- Agave nectar

The items that have the highest amounts are listed at the top, so don't be fooled by there being sugar in many different ingredients.

Sources of Sugar Cravings

Sugar itself is actually a very addictive food so you could wean yourself off of it gradually, as one method of getting rid of your cravings for it.

Additionally, you should consider whether or not you have an overgrowth of candida or parasites living in your gut in such numbers so as to be the biggest source of your sugar cravings. Both of these unwelcome living beings require large amounts of sugar to survive, and they make you obtain it for them.

If you have these critters living inside of you, calling the shots and making you crave sugar, pack on pounds, which puts you at risk for getting diabetes and other major health problems, you need to evict these unwelcome guests.

Obviously, it would be worth going through the unpleasant process that is necessary to get rid of candida or parasites because doing so would give you the control you need to keep diabetes out of your life.

It would be wise to get yourself a colonics board and flush a bunch of these critters out of your system before you get started with a program. Getting rid of the rest of candida or parasites by other methods later will go a bit easier if you get rid of the extras early on through irrigation.

You would then do well to continue to use your system monthly or at least bi-yearly for the rest of your life. As a benefit, you will feel better immediately after you do colonics.

Markus Rothkranz is a health guru. Here is his basic attack plan specifically for getting rid of parasites:

1. Flush out what you can get out easily using a colonic board. If you can't afford to buy one, get yourself an enema bag.

2. Starve the hangers-on by going on a one-month vegetable juice fast and consuming no source of sugar or carbohydrates. Craving for sugar will be fierce but fight this craving. It will eventually go away as the worms weaken and/or die.

3. Evict the weakened worms with special parasite herbs.

4. Make the larvae and the eggs unwelcome also by keeping up with the limited diet and taking the herbs.

5. Flush out what you can as you go through these weeks.

You will gain many health benefits by doing colonics, but the main goal for you as a reader of a book about diabetes is to avoid diabetes, control diabetes, or reverse diabetes. It is a goal worth fighting for, and *fight you will* when you get to the stage that you starve off these unwelcome guests who demand more and more sugar. You will crave the junk food like you never have for a while.

Ultimately, though, you will reclaim your general health, get rid of the cravings and set yourself on a healthy path, away from a future with diabetes.

Candida, in particular, is a common reason for massive weight gain. If you think you may have candida, talk to an allergy specialist. He can tell you whether or not you have candida overgrowth. If you suffer from food allergies and/or another kind of allergies, you may have candida because candida is often present when a person suffers from allergies.

To get rid of candida, the allergy doctor will prescribe Nystatin or some other medication that will kill the candida. Since you want the drug to kill off the candida, consult your allergy doctor about if and when to do colonics while on a candida program.

Both candida and parasite overgrowth adversely affect health in many areas. I won't go into them here, but you can easily find information about them on the internet. You won't find many general practitioners informing patients about them. They make more money on prescribing medications for symptoms.

Choose Fats Wisely

We often think of fat as bad, but there are types of fat that have a lot of health benefits. One just needs to eat the healthy fats.

Unhealthy fats – Artificial trans fats are the worst kind of fats. They exist in commercially-baked goods, fried food, packaged snack food, and in anything that is labeled "partly hydrogenated," even if claiming to be free of trans fats.

Healthy fats – You want unsaturated fats. They can be found in fish and in plants such as nuts, avocados, and olive oil. Salmon, tuna, and flaxseeds also contain omega-3 fatty acids, which support the heart and the brain. They also fight inflammation.

Saturated fats – You would be okay to enjoy these in moderation, as in no more than 10% of the diet, according to the American Diabetes Association. Saturated fats are found in red meat, tropical oils, and dairy.

Note: Organic coconut oil is a saturated fat. It is not a Western kind of food, so it is just now reaching the mainstream news in the West. It must be taken in smaller quantities, such as between two and four tablespoons per day, however, because it can cause diarrhea in some people.

Organic coconut oil lowers blood sugar, which is great news for diabetics who love sweets. Replacement of longer chain polyunsaturated fats with saturated fat such as coconut oil can reduce your cravings for refined carbs, which contribute to insulin resistance.

Organic coconut oil also reverses dementia in many people in a pretty short period of time. With all of this good news, coconut oil is one of the best kept dietary secrets ever kept!

To take control of your fat intake, you will:

- Stop eating chips and crackers
- Stop frying food
- Stop buying processed meat
- Stop buying packaged meals
- Stop buying takeout food
- Stop eating mainly red meat
- Stop buying commercial salad dressings
- Eat fewer dairy items

- Start snacking on nuts, seeds, and nut butter
- Broil, bake, and stir-fry
- Eat much more chicken, fish, eggs
- Eat much more protein that comes from vegetables
- Use extra virgin olive oil (cold-pressed) in pasta dishes, to cook veggies with and to put into salads.
- Create your own salad dressings using flaxseed, sesame seed, or extra virgin olive oil.
- Put sliced avocados into salads and sandwiches
- Consume more organic or raw cheese, milk, butter and yogurt

Tips Regarding Alcohol Consumption

Alcohol is not actually off limits for a diabetic unless your doctor tells you otherwise. In fact, research has actually shown that alcohol reduces the risk for heart disease. It just needs to be consumed in a moderate amount, such as no more than one drink per day for women and two for men. One drink is the equivalent of one 12 oz. beer or 5 oz. a glass of wine or 1.5 oz. distilled spirits.

There are additional rules for the diabetic, however, when it comes to drinking alcohol. They are:

- Do not drink when your blood sugar is low or on an empty stomach. Drink with your meal. This is especially important for people who are on insulin or diabetes pills which lower insulin.
- Don't count alcohol as a carbohydrate.
- Wear an ID bracelet or something that lets people know you have diabetes.
- Drink slowly.
- Hydrate yourself with a zero-calorie drink such as water or tea.
- Try a wine spritzer made with wine or a light beer with ice cubes and a club soda. Beware of alcohol-laden craft beers.
- For mixed drinks, use zero-calorie drink mixers such as tonic water, diet soda or water.

- Do not drive after you drink for several hours.
- Check your blood sugar level before you go to bed. It needs to be between 100 and 140 mg/dL. Eat something if it is too low.

You need to realize that the symptoms of hypoglycemia and too much alcohol can be similar. Those symptoms include dizziness, sleepiness, and disorientation. The only way emergency medical people can know how to help you if you are hypoglycemic rather than drunk is to wear ID jewelry that says, "I have diabetes." Also, don't let your alcohol consumption deter you from your meal plan.

Eat Regularly and Keep a Food Diary

There is no need to starve yourself. You don't need to count calories either when attempting to drastically cut your risk of getting diabetes. What seems to be doable to most people is to 1) eat on a regular eating schedule and 2) record what you eat.

Eat at regular times. Your body regulates sugar levels and your weight better when it get nutrition on a schedule.

Eat a healthy breakfast. A good breakfast will make your blood sugar levels steadier and give you energy throughout your morning.

Eat up to six small meals throughout the day. This will keep your proportions small.

Eat the same number of calories from day to day. Keeping the daily calorie count the same from day to day helps to regulate blood sugar levels. Don't binge one day and starve the next.

Keep a food diary. This is the biggest factor in losing weight because you identify problem areas, such as the what, why and how much you're eating. You will begin to eat less of the stuff that keeps you fat and start eating quality food.

Chapter 4: Prevent/Treat/Reverse Diabetes with Edible Plants

Free food and medicine are growing all around us, but modern people, for the most part, have little knowledge of this fact. Modern people in the Western world trust the medical establishment, which offers them conventional Western solutions. The patients endure the high costs, inconvenience, and pain of managing diabetes rather than preventing it, treating it or even reversing it with healthy food, including edible plants.

This is not how the man was meant to live. In fact, it is a step backward from how readily our ancestors treated ailments. Some of the diseases we consider common weren't even known in earlier times because people ate more wholesome food and had not yet been introduced to diseases from other lands.

The medicinal plants that are of use in the fight against diabetes come in the form of berries, daisy-like flowers, dandelion-like plants, desert plants, flowers, grasses, herbs, seaweed, trees, umbrella flowers, and in Uncategorized types all their own.

You can grow much of this "pharmacy" in your own back yard. The rest can be ordered online or perhaps found locally, depending on where you live. Over time, you can gradually cut back on their prescription meds, under the doctor's approval, of course.

Edible Plants Containing Diabetes-Fighting Properties

Berries – Currant, Goji, Grape, Huckleberry, Kiwi, Raspberry Leaves, Schizandra

Daisy-Like Flowers –	Daisy Fleabane
Dandelion-Like –	Dandelion
Desert Plants -	Aloe Vera, Cape Aloe, Chapparal, Prickly Pear Cactus
Flowers –	Begonia, Bluets, Evening Primrose, Jerusalem Artichoke, Marshmallow
Grasses –	Alfalfa
Herbs -	Balsam Pear, Bugleweed, Cayenne, Chanca Piedra, Chili Pepper, Coleus Forskohlii, Coral Vine, Fenugreek, Garlic, Gentian, Ginseng, Goat's Rue, Green Tea, Heal-All, Kudzu, Licorice-Wild, Nettle, Olive, Onion, Oregano, Sage, Sumac-Smooth, Solomon's Seal, Stevia, Uva Ursi, Yellow Root
Seaweed –	Kelp
Trees –	Almond, Avacado, Cedar Berries, Cinnamon, Juniper Berries, Kumquat, Loquat, Moringa, Mullberry, Prickly Ash
Umbrella Flowers –	Carrot-Wild, Parsley, Yarrow
Uncategorized –	Lecithin, Pomegranate, Squash, Watercress

Here are the same plants with a little more detail.

BERRIES:

Currant – Related to gooseberries, this shrub grows to a height of two to four feet high and bears red, white or black berries. The blackberries cluster in groups of four to six berries. The leaves resemble those of maples leaves.

Goji – This berry is a member of the nightshades family and resembles the poisonous Bittersweet Berry. Both have purple flowers. Goji is used for diabetes, but there currently is no official proof of its effectiveness in combating diabetes. Eat Goji raw, dry, juiced, blended or in tea.

Grape-Wild - Wild black, green, red, purple and white clusters of grapes grow everywhere. Plant a tiny grape plant, or even a cutting from another plant. It will grow fast and provide you with a lifetime of food. Eat the berries raw, blended into smoothies or juiced. Eat the leaves as wraps.

Huckleberry - Huckleberries are related to blueberries. Their colors range from blue-purple to red to almost black, and each berry contains 10 large hard seeds. Their stems are smooth, and the leaves have small yellow dots on the underside.
Eat as you would eat blueberries.

Kiwi – This fuzzy little fruit grows vigorously on a vine. The fruit looks like hairy brown eggs. Eat them raw, including the hairy skin.

Raspberry Leaves – The raspberries are nutritious, but the left gives nutrition that the berries do not. The plant produces berries three times per year. The leaves appear early in the spring and stay until a cold frost. Make tea from the leaves

Schizandra – This plant grows anywhere, but it originated from China. Dry the berries and make into powder or make into tea. The leaves and the roots can also be consumed. Do not consume if you are pregnant.

DAISY-LIKE FLOWERS:

Daisy Fleabane – These daisy-like flowers have pinkish lavender flowers that are yellowish in the middle of them. Consume the whole plant for tea.

DANDELION-LIKE:

Dandelion – The dandelion is a part of the lettuce family, and they have a yellow flower on top. The entire plant is edible, even the milk sap in the stems, but the leaves need to be eaten when they are young.

DESERT PLANTS:

Aloe Vera – This cactus heals itself whenever it is cut. It knows the difference between normal cells and diseased cells and stops diseased cells from spreading.

Cape Aloe – This cactus came to the United States from South Africa and now grows in the southwestern part of the U.S. It can grow to be 12 feet high! Do not take if pregnant.

Chapparal – There are more than 20 species of this plant. These plants can survive the scorching desert heat and live to be 25,000 years old! Do not consume chapparal fresh. You need to dry it dry out for a couple of months, then grind the dried leaves into a powder that you put into juice or water to drink. Do not consume if you are pregnant.

Prickly Pear Cactus - The plant grows all over the world.

All of the plants can be consumed. This cactus has pink fruit on it, which can be eaten. The fruit tastes like raspberries. You can make tea from the pads of the plant or put the whole thing into a high-powered blender such as the Vitamix to put into smoothies.

FLOWERS:

Begonia – This is a common house plant which has many varieties which are edible. Although the entire plant is edible, the flowers are consumed to help with diabetes.

Bluets – These are small blue, violet or white flowers that have four petals and a yellow center.

Evening Primrose – These plants grow to be four to five feet tall. They have yellow flowers that consist of four petals. The petals open at night and close during the day. The flowers grow on the branches. Use them in stir-fry or casserole dishes. The whole plant is edible. Harvest the seed pods before they flower and treat them like okra.

Jerusalem Artichoke – These are related to sunflowers and are not artichokes. These grow to be almost nine feet tall. And have yellow flowers. Eat the roots of these after the first frost. Eat throughout the winter. You can put these in salads or steamed. Can use the juice from the roots as a sugar substitute since it is sweet.

Marshmallow – The leaves can be eaten in salads. Avoid the roots since they are high in sugar.

GRASSES:

Alfalfa – This grass has a flowered clover of purple color and roots the reach over 100 feet deep. Dry the grass, then grind it into a powder. Make tea with it, juice it, or put it into smoothies. Eat only a little of it if you have lupus.

HERBS:

Balsam Pear – This is a smelly plant. Do not eat if you are pregnant or trying to get pregnant. Do not eat this plant raw except for the seed covers. Spit the seeds out. When this plant is turning from green to red, do not eat the outer shell of the plant or the seeds, but you can eat the red fleshy seed covers, even raw. Do not eat it when they are orange and ripe either. Only eat or juice this when it is green and has been boiled twice. The whole thing, seeds and all can be eaten if boiled and the water is changed after the first boiling. This plant can drop blood sugar rapidly, so beware of it. Leaves are edible only if cooked and drained.

Bugleweed – The entire plant is edible, but it should not be eaten by people who have a hypothyroid condition.

Cayenne – Good for diabetics, but people with hypoglycemia should stay away from it. Taking this with anything else increases the absorption of the other herbs. Do not eat the flower part of this because they are nightshade.

Chanca Piedra - This plant is common in tropical areas. It grows up to two feet tall. Take as a tea, an extract, powder or put into capsules. It is suggested to drink one to two cups of tea per day on an empty stomach or else one teaspoon of the powder form put into the water three times per day.

Chili Peppers – Good for diabetic neuropathy. Like almost all of the other plants listed here, this one helps with many different ailments in addition to diabetes.

Coleus Forskohlii – This is a tropical perennial plant. It is also an ayurvedic herb that is from the mint/lavender family. Do not take this if you are on blood thinners. Oral hypoglycemics, high blood pressure medications, heart medications or if you have abnormally low blood pressure or a bleeding disorder.

Coral Vine – This plant is from the buckwheat family, and the vine grows very aggressively. Its seeds are shaped like pyramids, the leaves like hearts and the flowers are white or pink. The entire plant is edible, but the flowers and the leaves should be cooked or steamed. For diabetics, dry the leaves and make tea with them.

Fenugreek – The entire plant is edible. This seed lowers the glucose and insulin responses in diabetics that are not dependent on insulin. When toasted, this is a healthy sugar substitute that resembles the taste of maple syrup. It tastes bitter if eaten raw. This should not be eaten by pregnant women.

Garlic – This plant looks like grass with edible bulbs on top and has cloves underground. The bulbs and the cloves are edible, but to benefit from their nutrients, one needs to crush, dice, slice or ground them so as to break open the cells. There is a look-alike plant that is poisonous, so make sure you have garlic. You will know by its smell.

Gentian – There are more than 400 varieties of this plant, and their trumpet-shaped flowers come in white, yellow, blue or red.

Ginseng – This herb acts like insulin for sugar removal. Needs to be taken long-term to get noticeable effects.

Goat's Rue – This is a wild legume that has yellow and pink on its flowers. Helps to balance blood sugar levels

Green Tea – This evergreen provides endless tea. Use the young leaves and either boil them for 15 seconds or freeze them for 30 minutes. Then dry them to make tea with later. Don't drink all of the time, though, because it contains fluoride.

Heal-All – This herb from the mint family grows to be one to two feet tall and has white and purple cluster flowers and a reddish, square stem. All of the plants is edible. Put into salads or make tea with it.

Kudzu – This is an aggressively growing vine that has reddish purple flowers and hairy seedpods. It lowers blood sugar levels. The whole plant can be consumed.

Licorice-Wild – This wild version of licorice is similar to the Asian licorice root. Wild licorice can grow to be nine feet tall! It has small white flowers and prickly seed pods. This plant balances the blood sugar so the insulin levels can get cut over time with the guidance of a doctor. It is best to consume this plant for a month and then get off of it for a week or so and go back to it. Do not eat it if you have a history of renal failure or liver disease. Do not take if you are on heart medication or steroid drugs. Do not take if you are pregnant. Avoid the store-bought standardized form. You need this in its natural form.

Nettle – Stinging Nettle has jagged leaves with hairs on the underside that sting you if you touch it with your bare hands. There are also seeds on the stems. This plant increases insulin sensitivity and lowers the blood sugar levels. It can be injected in its natural state or made into a tea that can be put on the body externally for various reasons other than diabetes. The seeds can be ground into flour and made into pancakes, porridge or cereal. Sprout it in the winter. The only known species of nettle that is too strong to use grows in New Zealand and Australia, and it is called Urtica Ferox.

Olive – The curing process for olives takes three months. Most commercially available olives have been soaked in sodium hydroxide, which you don't want to eat, and the canned black ones have been soaked in ferrous gluconate, which is also bad for you. Olive oil that has been stone crushed is the best option for you. Most cold pressed olive oil has been heated so high that they kill the life force in the olives.

Onion – Onion is good for many ailments, including diabetes. Make sure you are eating an onion and not a poisonous look-alike.

Oregano – This plant is in the mint family, and it has pinkish purple flowers. Fresh wild oregano is a powerful plant that slows down complications associated with diabetes. This plant can be eaten and applied topically. If you are taking probiotics, do not take oregano because it kills the good bacteria. Put two to three drops of oregano oil under the tongue three times daily for three days and then take probiotics.

Sage – This is another member of the mint family. It has red, white, blue, pink or purple flowers. Sage boosts insulin production. Eat sage leaves every day.

Sumac-Smooth – This plant grows to be from three to twenty feet high and produces hairy berries. The whole plant is usable, and all of it controls diabetes, but you want to eat the berries when they are red, not white. The berries can be chewed or made into tea. Soak the fruit and make lemonade. You'll need to eat the shoots when they are young. You can eat the roots peeled and raw. Eat the flowers, fruit, bark and the leaves too.

Solomon's Seal – This plant has drooping branches that are laden with yellow, green and white flowers. To treat diabetes, bake the roots in the sun or boil with three changes of water and then make into tea. Do not eat the berries.

Stevia – This is sugar that you can have, as it has no effect on the pancreas, insulin or blood sugar other than to regulate the diabetic's blood sugar and help with diabetic cataracts and impotence. It is therefore safe for diabetics. It helps the body to absorb whatever else is eaten with it.

Uva Ursi – This is a low-growing shrub that only grows to be a few inches tall. It has fine hairy bark, pink or white flowers, red berries and shiny leaves that look like plastic. It lowers excessive sugar in the blood. Do not take this longer than a week or you will damage your liver. Do not take it if you are pregnant or have kidney disease. Do not give to children.

Yellow Root – This small shrub was appropriately named after its yellow roots. It also has yellow bark. It has brown-purple flowers that droop. Make a tea from the roots to treat diabetes.

SEAWEED:

Parsley – Grow this plant next to asparagus, roses and other garden plants to keep the bugs away

Yarrow – This plant grows to be about two feet tall. Its flowers
Kelp – This is protein from the sea. This plant helps with both weight loss, strengthens the heart, and helps treat diabetes, among many things.

TREES:

Almond – Almonds are actually seeds rather than nuts, and they are something you could live off of if you had to because they are highly nutritious and contain almost all of the things the body needs. The outer fleshy part can be eaten and is at its best when the fruit is still young before the insides harden.

Avocado – This fruit is high in monounsaturated fat, which is good. The pit is rich in minerals and can be liquefied in a high-powered blender such as the Vitamix. The leaves, however, are toxic.

Cedar Berries – Cedar trees grow to be 10 to 20 feet high. They resemble juniper, but cedars have one large blue-green berry stone with little flesh instead of three to seven stones like the Juniper has. Cedar berries help diabetics to cut down on insulin. Do not consume if pregnant, and do not consume cedar oil ever.

Cinnamon – This tree grows to be 50 feet tall. Cinnamon, which comes from the bark, stabilizes blood sugar.

Juniper Berry – Not all of the more than 50 varieties of juniper are edible, but the most edible variety of juniper is Juniperus Communis. Consume the berries only after they have turned purple in color, not when they are still green. Be aware that it takes some berries three years to ripen. Boil juniper needles to make tea. Smash and consume just a few berries at a time. Do not consume if you are pregnant.

Kumquat – These shrubby looking trees only grow to be 15 feet tall. They have white citrus flowers, and their leaves are dark, glossy and pointed, as fruit tree leaves normally are. Their orang-yellow fruit is like oranges that are the size of grapes and can be eaten whole like grapes. The juice on the inside of the fruit is sour, but the rind/peel is sweet. The peeling part of the fruit is what is beneficial to diabetics.

Loquat –This tree grows up to 30 feet tall. It has leathery leaves, sweet-smelling white flowers, and delicious yellow-orange fruit. Great for diabetics.

Moringa – This is a popular tree that grows to be nine feet tall in its first 10 months of life and reaches heights up 30 feet tall. It loves the sun and hates frost. It is often planted in people's gardens and is used for food and medicine in developing countries. For diabetics, the plant stabilizes blood sugar levels All parts of the tree are used. The roots grow very deep into the ground, and they taste like horseradish. The leaves are used to make stir-fry, stews, salads, tea, and soup. Young seedpods are edible, as are the mature seeds and the flowers. All of the tree, including the bark, has medicinal value, but the leaves offer the most nutrition. The leaves are used like spinach, so they are eaten raw, cooked, put into soup, or are dried and made into powder. Eat the seeds like peas or roast them like nuts.

Mulberry – Male and female trees are required for a tree to bear fruit, and the delicious berries are what the diabetic needs. The leaves, however, do not break down carbohydrates to simple sugars. Berries taste great if dried and then ground down and mixed with ground nuts, made into candy balls.

Prickly Ash – The northern prickly ash trees grow to be 30 feet in height, while the southern version grows to be 45 feet in height. Both have sharp thorns sticking out of the branches and the trunks. The bark is used as a stimulant, preventing the constriction of blood vessels by insulin.

UMBRELLA FLOWERS:

Carrot, Wild – Wild carrot grows biannually, and there is not much difference between them and what you would find in a grocery store.
come in various colors, and they resemble daisies. Dry the entire plant and use as tea.

UNCATEGORIZED:

Lecithin – You will have to get this from a supplement. It is found in the cell membranes, and it is created in the liver from dietary choline.

Pomegranate – Pomegranate improves the blood flow to the heart and decreases the artery plaque while not affecting the blood glucose level in diabetics.

Squash – This is a good item for diabetics to eat.

Watercress – This one is a strong medicine that is used for many different ailments. You will find these living close to water.

Edible Plants That Combat Diabetic Retinopathy

Berries –	Bilberry, Schizandra
Desert Plants –	Aloe Vera, Cape Aloe
Herbs –	Garlic, Sage
Trees –	Juniper, Pine Bark
Uncategorized –	Pomegranate

BERRIES:

Bilberry – This berry is similar to blueberries, but these berries are red or purple throughout. Protects against diabetes by strongly lowering blood sugar. Dry the berries and the leaves, then make tea out of it.

Schizandra – This plant grows anywhere, but it originated from China. Dry the berries and make into powder or make into tea. The leaves and the roots can also be consumed. Do not consume if you are pregnant.

DESERT PLANTS:

Aloe Vera – This cactus heals itself whenever it is cut. It can even tell the difference between normal cells and diseased cells, which it stops from spreading.

Cape Aloe – This cactus came to the United States from South Africa and now grows in the southwestern part of the U.S. It can grow to be 12 feet high! Do not take if pregnant.

HERBS:

Garlic – This plant looks like grass with edible bulbs on top and has cloves underground. The bulbs and the cloves are edible, but to benefit from their nutrients, one needs to crush, dice, slice or ground them so as to break open the cells. There is a look-alike plant that is poisonous, so make sure you have garlic. You will know by its smell.

Sage – This is another member of the mint family. It has red, white, blue, pink or purple flowers. Sage boosts insulin production. Eat sage leaves every day.

TREES:

Juniper Berry – Not all of the more than 50 varieties of juniper are edible, but the most edible variety of juniper is Juniperus Communis. Consume the berries only after they have turned purple in color, not when they are still green. Be aware that it takes some berries three years to ripen. Boil juniper needles to make tea. Smash and consume just a few berries at a time. Do not consume if you are pregnant.

Pine Bark – Pine bark protects the arterial system and improves circulation as it supports diabetes.

UNCATEGORIZED:

Pomegranate – This item improves the blood flow to the heart and decreases artery plaque, but it does not affect the blood glucose levels in diabetics.

Chapter 5: Prevent/Treat/Reverse Diabetes with Physical Activity

Exercise lowers blood glucose in two ways:

1. During and after physical activity, your insulin sensitivity is increased. That makes your cells better able to use the insulin during that time.

2. A different mechanism is stimulated when your muscles contract that helps your cells to use the glucose for energy, whether or not insulin is available.

Exercise lowers blood sugar in the short-term in these two ways, keeping your blood glucose lower for somewhere around 24 hours. How long you benefit from exercise depends on several factors, though. If you are active on a regular basis, your hemoglobin A1C is also lowered.

It would be helpful to you if you come to know how your blood glucose responds to exercise. You need to 1) check your blood glucose level before and after exercise, and 2) test different types of exercise to see how your body responds. Doing these two things will let you know what your physical exercise routine should be.

Whether you have Type 1 diabetes or Type 2 diabetes, you should be prepared to treat yourself for hypoglycemia. However, Type 1 diabetics are at the highest risk of becoming hypoglycemic. Type 2 diabetics may have an issue with it if they are on an insulin secretagogue or on insulin.

Treat hypoglycemia in the following way:

1. Consume at least 15-20 grams of a sugary food, such as glucose tabs, soda, or a sports drink. It would be more convenient to have glucose tablets with you at all times. You may not be so lucky as to have a person with you to go get you a drink or something if you have trouble.

2. Wait around 15 to 20 minutes. Then check your blood sugar again.

3. If nothing has improved, repeat the above process.

4. To continue exercising, take a break so as to treat your blood sugar. This depends on how much insulin you are running on and what you are doing for exercise.

5. If you stop exercising, make sure your blood sugar has come back up to above 100 mg/dl before you start to exercise again.

6. Eat regular meals and snacks once you feel better.

It is important to remember that your blood sugar can drop long after you exercise. It isn't just during exercise that this can happen to you. There are a few scenarios in which you can expect to have a hypoglycemic episode, which are:

1. You take your insulin.

2. You take your insulin secretagogue.

3. You skip a meal

4. You don't eat within a half hour or more after you stop exercising.

5. You exercise for a lengthy period of time.

6. Your exercise workout was strenuous.

If hypoglycemia becomes a frequent problem, talk to your doctor. He may adjust your treatment plan and/or he may tell you to eat a small snack before you exercise. If a long period of exercise is expected, both of these measures would need to be taken.

Extra carbohydrates will not be needed unless you plan to exercise for long periods of time. If you want to lose weight, just eat extra food just before you exercise.

Otherwise, it is important for you to focus on filling your plate with lean meat, healthy fats, low- or non-fat dairy, whole grains, fruit and non-starchy vegetables.

Chapter 6: Treat Your Feet

While you manage your diabetes with food choices, weight loss, and physical activity, it is also a good idea to take care of your feet. Infection can become a problem for people with diabetes, so proper care of them is necessary.

Foot problems include plantar warts, ingrown toenails, hammertoes, foot ulcers, dry skin, bunions, blisters, corns, fungal infections, calluses, athlete's foot, diabetic neuropathy and peripheral vascular disease.

Extreme diabetes-related foot problems can result in amputation, so it is important to watch for foot problems at the same time as you tackle the weight, diet and exercise aspects of treating diabetes.

Here are some good tips to follow when it comes to proper foot care:

- Follow your regular diabetic plan for food choices, exercise, etc., so as to keep the blood sugar level.
- Check your feet for the various types of foot problems, especially if you have poor blood circulation.
- Put lotion on your feet after you wash and dry them so that they never get cracks in the skin. Your doctor can tell you what brands to use.
- After you bathe, smooth down your corns and calluses, moving the emery board in one direction.
- Check your toenails weekly. Trim them straight across instead of rounding off at the corners. Smooth them with a file after clipping.
- Wear closed-toes shoes at all times when not sleeping.
- Don't wear shoes that have foreign objects in them.
- Stop smoking. Smoking worsens blood circulation problems.
- Contact your doctor for chronic foot problems.
- Have your diabetes doctor check your feet for sensation, temperature and skin problems.

-   Have a podiatrist also. Visit him every two or three months, even if you don't think you have a problem with your feet.

A diabetic needs to visit their doctor if they notice any one or more of the following symptoms:

-   Skin color changes
-   Skin temperature changes
-   Foot or ankle swelling
-   Leg pain
-   Draining or slow-healing open sores on feet
-   Infected or ingrown toenails
-   Corns or calluses
-   Dry cracks in heels or elsewhere
-   Persistent and/or unusual foot odor

Chapter 7: Recipes for Fruits and Vegetables

You can make up your own recipes as you go, even adding various wild edibles into vegetable salads, fruit salads, and smoothies that you customize to taste. You don't have to feel deprived of sweets either because you can learn to make things with coconut oil. As you read in the previous chapter, coconut oil actually lowers blood sugar levels and is therefore good for diabetics.

Always remember to include dark leafy items at some point in your day. Your body will tell you what it needs, so listen to it.

Here are a few recipe samples. You can make things up as you go, which is why there are few amounts listed, but you'll get the idea.

Mango Blueberry Mint (Salad)

Mango
Blueberries
Fresh mint leaves
Fresh chopped ginger
Chopped jalapeno pepper
Sea salt
Lime juice

Kale Salad (Salad, make with whatever sounds good)

Radishes
Red pepper
Onion
Avocado
Cucumber
Sprouts
Kale

Hot pepper
Finely chopped garlic
Sea salt

Dressing for the Kale Salad

1/3 fresh squeezed orange juice
1/3 Nama Shoyu
Olive oil to taste

Mix dressing in with the salad and let soak in the refrigerator for one hour. This softens the kale.

Avocado with Tropical Salsa (Salad)

Apple cider vinegar
Olive oil
Red onion
Papaya
Mango
Avocado
Cilantro
Pepper
Sea salt

Spicy Thai Cabbage (Salad)

Raisins
Raw cashew nuts
Scallions
Red cabbage
Sea salt
Cilantro

Dressing for Thai Cabbage

Sesame oil
Hot chili oil
Apple cider vinegar

Raw nut butter

Silicon Salad

Leaf lettuce, red
Onion
Nopales (cactus)
Cucumber
Okra

Dressing for Silicon Salad

Orange juice
Nama Shoyu
Olive oil

Directions: Shake the nuts in a bag with sea salt, agave nectar, and cayenne. Also, add the okra and the cactus just before serving because the silica in them makes them slimy after an hour.

Raw Fruit Pie (No baking/cooking)

Blueberries
Agave nectar
Vanilla
Lemon juice
Cashews
Coconut oil
Sea salt

Directions: Make the crust out of the dates and nuts. Mix everything else together, putting most of the fruit on the top. It looks like a cream cheese pie, and these are now available in many health food stores.

Raw Chocolate

Raw agave nectar
Raw nut butter
Raw carob powder
Cacao beans
Peppermint oil
Coconut oil
Vanilla

Directions: Grind the beans into a powder. Mix everything together. Chill.

Okay, so maybe you are wondering how to put dandelion weeds, bitter tasting things, and other weird-tasting things into something that you would deem tasty enough to eat. Well, you will want to just blend things like that in a high-powered blender such as a Vitamix along with better tasting items. Bitters are very good for you if you didn't know. You can blend all of the more disagreeable items with sweeter things to make a very good-tasting and extremely healthy morning drink.

Below are some blender recipes that don't contain the wild food, but all you would have to do is add the ones you want to them.

Quick Meal (Vitamix smoothie recipe)

Celery
Little Nama Shoyu
Sprouts
Parsley
Asparagus
Pineapple
Red leaf lettuce or kale
Coconut water and the meat

<u>Super-Fast Blender Meal</u> 2 (Vitamix smoothie recipe)

Avocado
Coconut water
Red leaf lettuce
Parsley
Sea salt

Note: As always, you can add whatever else you want to, such as celery, apples, etc. You could put this into a bowl after it is blended if you want and top with cashew nuts.

Conclusion

Thank for making it through to the end of this book, let's hope it was informative and able to provide you with all of the tools that you will need to achieve your goals whatever they may be.

As modern people in Western culture stopped exercising, let themselves grow fat, and strayed from eating healthy natural food over the last few decades, the general health of people declined and diabetes, like many other ailments, became an epidemic.

The baby boomers have reached their retirement years now, and many of them have diabetes. Diabetes is a miserable disease to live with, and it can lead to amputation of limbs, kidney failure, and dialysis treatments, heart problems and other things if it is not caught early, managed and/or reversed in time.

Healthcare is in a crisis situation in the United States, however, and treatment for diabetes is too expensive for seniors and others to afford. With all of the problems associated with diabetes and the outlandish costs of prescription medications, it is worth looking into the notion of returning to nature with the intent of deliberately eating the natural foods that are known to have positive effects on diabetes.

First of all, though, one needs to take the weight off. Concentrate on the abdomen area if that is where your weight likes to pile on. That mainly involves not eating certain foods, so it costs you nothing to get that area flattened. You will need to consult the book to know what specific abdomen-expanding foods to avoid.

Fit exercise into your daily routine, as well as your healthy meals. You may want to plant yourself a pharmacy garden that contains some of the listed edible plants that combat diabetes.

When you start to eat a good amount of your homegrown food, you will need to have your doctor test you to see whether or not

he needs to adjust your insulin medication. You don't want to
have too much insulin!

Finally, if you found this book useful in any way, please review it
on Amazon. It would be appreciated!